CONTENTS

INTRODUCTION TO THE PALEO DIET

WHAT IS THE PALEO DIET?

The Paleo diet is considered a primal or "caveman" diet, because it focuses on food options that were around during ancient times, before farming and the cultivation of crops was developed.

Principles of the Paleo Diet

Before you begin adapting to the paleo way of eating, it's important to understand the principles of the reasoning behind the food choices and meal options available. There are some basics to become familiar with when you begin, to have a good foundation of understanding:

- This diet includes foods in their most natural, unprocessed state, without any preservatives or additives. In adhering to these parameters, you'll avoid hidden sugars, artificial sweeteners, and over-processed boxed and packaged foods.
- Plant-based options are entirely fresh or frozen, often avoiding canned as an option, due to the high level of

preservatives often included. Dried fruit and vegetable chips are a great option, though best as homemade.

- Foods associated with cultivation, such as grains, legumes, and beans are avoided, as they do not fit within the primal options of food that paleo includes. Since farming wasn't developed during ancient primal times, these foods are generally avoided.

- High carbohydrate foods like rice, grains, and pasta are skipped, and instead, the focus is on root vegetables and organic fruits for a better carb option. Paleo doesn't specifically limit or avoid carbohydrates, though it focuses on natural, organic foods that contain high-quality carbs, which make a significant impact on the nutritional value of your meals.

- Nuts and seeds are strong staples in the paleo diet and cater to many variations of this way of eating, including plant-based and low carb. They are best consumed in their natural form, without any sugar, sodium, or flavoring added.

- All meat, specifically lean cuts of beef, pork, chicken, and turkey, are included in the paleo diet. Fish is an excellent option for including healthy fats, protein, and calcium. Game meats such as venison, are also a welcome inclusion in this way of eating.

- Dairy is not generally included, especially in strict Paleo diets; however, some may include small amounts.

Consider the types of foods our ancestors had access to thousands of years ago, before farming, cultivation, and processing. During those times, you ate what you could find or forage for, and the animals you hunted. This was a simple and effective way of feeding yourself, family, and community. Food wasn't necessarily cooked or prepared in any way, but enjoyed in its complete and natural state, whether it was raw meat, fish, berries, root vegetables, leaves, insects and other forms of animals and vegetation, depending on the region and the climate.

The Benefits of Adapting to the Paleo Way of Eating

What are the advantages of following a Paleo diet? There are plenty of reasons to adapt to this way of eating, and understanding the specific benefits can be a major reason to make the change. The impact of the paleo method will have a significant effect on your physical and mental health. The following advantages are common in many people who adapt to the paleo method:

Weight Loss

One of the most common reasons for adhering to the paleo diet is weight loss, and the ability to maintain a healthy weight for the long-term. The high fiber and nutrient content ensure your body receives a balanced diet complete with just the right amounts of natural sugar, sodium, and healthy fats, without excessive amounts of any content. The paleo diet's carb content tends to range from low to moderate, depending on the types of vegetables and fruits chosen for meal preparation and planning. Studies conducted on the results of participants following a paleo diet indicate consist of weight loss with significant improvement within a short period. Consistent weight loss results are a positive sign of the effects that the Paleo diet has on your body and metabolic function in general.

Muscle Gain and Healthier Bones

If losing muscle density is a concern, paleo will increase and keep your bones and muscles strong and healthy for the duration of your lifetime. In addition to containing adequate levels of vitamin C, A, and E, which aid in the absorption of vitamin D, your body will have sufficient amounts of calcium and protein. Together, these nutrients ensure your bones and cartilage remain healthy and strong, preventing deterioration of the spine and vertebrae as you age. Following the elements of Paleo can help prevent osteoporosis and arthritis, among other conditions that are related to age and degeneration.

A Better Night's Rest

Insomnia will soon become a thing of the past, as you experience an improved quality of sleep and more of it. You'll toss and turn less and be able to "crash" sooner and feel refreshed in the morning. Better sleep is the result of a nutrient-rich diet full of organic and whole foods. It's important to understand that whether or not you can have all the hours of sleep you need, this is no guarantee that the quality will be adequate. For example, some people complain about not feeling well-rested, even if they have been in bed for 7-8 hours in total. Chances are, they did not sleep completely during the night, or experienced several interruptions and issues that prevented them from good rest. If you have a lot on your mind, stress or other factors can disrupt good rest, making it difficult to maintain consistent sleep, and avoiding REM (rapid eye movement) or deep sleep.

Stronger Mental Focus and Clarity

A diet high in natural, organic foods without preservatives will improve your brain's health, protecting you against many cognitive diseases and memory loss. Consuming Paleo foods will strengthen your brain's health for decades, including in your mature years.

Healthier Insulin and Blood Glucose Levels

Most Paleo foods are low in carbs, which makes them a better choice for people who are at risk for diabetes and high blood sugar. Carbohydrates are converted into glucose once they are ingested and absorbed, which quickly spikes sugar levels in the body, forcing the pancreas to produce more insulin. This can eventually lead to the development of type 2 diabetes, which can lead to other conditions and medical challenges later in life. By reducing the carbohydrates that you consume, the resistance to insulin is reduced also, which prevents the risk of type 2 diabetes. If you are already diagnosed with diabetes, reducing both your sugar and carb intake will greatly improve your health and prognosis for the future.

Improved Gut Health

Your gut's lining and bacteria will be more balanced, promoting better digestion and microbial balance within your body. Fermented foods are excellent for promoting good digestion, such as kimchi and sauerkraut, both of which are Paleo-friendly and easy to enjoy with a variety of meals, from roast beef, pork chops, chicken or baked salmon, as an example. Sauerkraut is a traditional German dish that is made by fermenting cabbage. Kimchi is a Korean fermented dish that is often spicy and created using cabbage, radishes, or other vegetables. While these fermented foods are great side dishes, they are also ideal as a light meal or snack as well.

Mental Health Benefits

Eating Paleo can reduce the symptoms and effects of depression, anxiety, and related conditions. The natural sugar balance occurs when you avoid processed ingredients, foods, and refined sweeteners and sugars, which can negatively change moods to change erratically and without notice. If you suffer from a mood disorder, you will benefit from Paleo's balanced approach to eating balanced and highly nutritious meals. Studies have indicated the positive effect that nutrient-dense foods have on your cognitive function and the ability to cope with a variety of conditions. While medical treatment may be necessary, eating well will improve the quality of your life and help you achieve a balance.

Increased Energy and Endurance

When you consume natural foods, your body will thrive and reward you with a higher level of energy, as well as endurance. If you plan on joining a marathon or another high-intensity exercise or goal, eating Paleo will take you to the finish line with a sense of renewed energy and satisfaction. By avoiding the high consumption of sugar and foods high in the glycemic index, you can avoid the "crash" that often follows after eating a sweet pastry or another sweetener-filled treat. The amount of natural sugar we need in our diet can be found naturally in fruits and other foods in their whole state, including some vegetables. A sustainable and long-lasting source of energy can be achieved by eating lean sources of protein from lean meats and plant-based foods. As your body utilizes protein sources, muscle tissue is built and strengthened, which lasts far longer than sugar, which is a temporary form of energy, which falls short of any long-term benefits or goals. Endurance is achieved by steadily eating balanced, natural foods as part of the Paleo diet. As you consume more foods high in natural energy, such as fiber, protein, and nutrients, you'll experience a better outcome in all of your physical endeavors and goals.

Reduced Inflammation

Since the Paleo diet has little to not acidic-producing foods, which are often the culprit for inflammation, which is also a side effect of chronic illness and eating foods high in sugar and carbohydrates. The balanced, alkaline-based foods part of the Paleo diet assure that you will not suffer from inflammation due to the low glycemic levels and moderate to high levels of omega 3s, 6s and healthy fats included in this way of eating.

In general, the Paleo diet has plenty of benefits for everyone, and can easily fit into any lifestyle, due to the variety of foods available. It is important to focus on the quality and choice of the foods and ingredients you choose, as opposed to the calories or carbohydrate count, as with many other diets. This type of focus on nutrition means you'll enjoy a higher quality in the meals you consume, along with the reduced sugar, unnatural and refined ingredients, while simply enjoying the foods you choose as a part of your regular eating habits.

BEGINNING THE PALEO DIET

TAKING the First Steps to a Cleaner, Natural Way of Eating

If you're new to the Paleo diet, there are some significant changes to make in the way you eat and choose your food. This can take time and will likely not occur overnight. It's recommended to start slowly by making subtle but meaningful changes that will make a difference over time. Some of the foods we eat may seem harmless, even beneficial if we are led to believe they are good for us. Years ago, campaigns were promoting the consumption of eight glasses of milk each day, without any consideration for allergic reactions and additives that can be found in some types of non-grass fed and processed forms of milk in the grocery stores. Plant-based diets have also received mixed reviews, and while the Paleo diet isn't completely based on vegan eating, it does involve many fresh fruits and vegetables as a significant part of the eating plan. The following two sections detail the most important foods to include in the Paleo diet, as well as the foods that should be avoided at all costs.

Top Foods for the Paleo Diet

There are many foods high in nutritional value that fit within the primal category of the paleo diet and can be included in a variety of meals and snacks. These foods are exemplary for their high nutritional value and provide a good source of nutrients for daily requirements. Consider including options from the following food choices below regularly, to fulfill your nutritional needs.

Dark Green Vegetables

Kale, spinach, and arugula are some of the most nutrient-dense vegetables to include in your daily meal plan to ensure you meet your daily requirements and avoid deficiencies. While all vegetables are highly nutritious, dark greens are strong in iron, calcium, multiple vitamins, and fiber content. As bitter as these vegetables are, they provide a decent base for salads, which can be naturally sweetened with citrus and/or maple syrup and berries. Spinach and arugula provide a good base for salads, or as a way to replace grains, such as rice, beans or pasta, with a serving of chicken, beef or seafood.

Nuts and Seeds

These are an important source of plant-based protein, calcium, and vitamins. Chia seeds contain some of the strongest seeds for nutrient value, with additional vitamins, antioxidants, and other benefits. They are often considered one of the "superfoods" which belong to a group of foods that provide an extremely dense serving of nutrients that can meet the daily requirements for certain vitamins in minerals in just one serving. Almonds, cashews, sesame seeds, sunflower and pumpkin seeds, among many other options, contain an abundance of healthy fats, protein, fiber, vitamins, and calcium. Some Paleo diet follows who prefer a more plant-based approach can find the required daily protein in a daily serving of nuts and/or seeds.

Bananas

A popular snack food, bananas receive special mention because they can provide a significant amount of benefits on their own, or in conjunction with other fruits. Just one banana can provide up to one and a half hours of energy. They not only contain fiber and vitamins but are also a good source of potassium, which helps to prevent inflammation and water retention. Bananas are excellent as a quick snack, and they can also be added to desserts or smoothies to create a tasty treat within a few minutes.

Root Vegetables

Turnips (rutabaga), potatoes, yams, beets, and other root-based vegetables are an excellent source of vitamins, and often provide a natural (unprocessed) form of carbohydrates. These vegetables are not only high in nutrients, but they are also pleasant in flavor and provide a filling side dish or as a main feature in plant-based meals. They are inexpensive and pair well with almost any other ingredients, including any other vegetables, meats, and spices. Carrots and parsnips are also excellent, tasty options to include in your next roast or skillet meal. All varieties of squash, including butternut, acorn, and spaghetti squash, are excellent sources of potassium and beta carotene. Root vegetables also contain a strong source of vitamins, and often enjoyed in a side dish or as part of dinner.

Lean Meats

Red meats such as beef and pork, as well as poultry, can be included in the Paleo diet. A moderate portion of meat is an excellent meal feature with a salad, soup, or baked vegetable. Highly nutritious bone broths, containing collagen, can be created from the bones of a leftover roast or meal. Often, beef and chicken broths are created, though this can be made from fish or other types of meat, including lamb, pork and other cuts of meat. Using meats in a variety of dishes is the best way to enjoy them, and many spices and seasonings can be applied to vary the taste each time. The best way to enjoy meat is to buy in bulk from a local butcher or market and freeze a large portion, using just enough for meals each day.

Seafood

Fish is an excellent source of protein, calcium, and healthy fats. These staple nutrients in a Paleo diet, as they can be found in many primitive food sources from hunting. Any variety of fish is good, and while some

Citrus Fruits

Oranges, lemons, limes, and grapefruit are strong sources of vitamin C and fiber. They tend to be acidic initially, though they become alkaline once ingested. The level of vitamins in these fruits are excellent for the prevention of the common cold and help support and build a stronger immune system. They are also refreshing in taste, whether you enjoy them as they are, include a splash of them in your water or sparkling beverage, or fruit or dark green salad. Grapefruit and oranges are excellent made into freshly squeezed juice, or as an addition to a breakfast meal. They make a wonderful snack during the day. Lemon and lime are often used in homemade dressings and vinaigrette mixes. They are often used in recipes for baking and puddings.

Apples

A strong alkaline food, apples are a good source of energy and vitamin C. They are convenient to enjoy on the go and make an excellent addition to the Paleo diet. Apples are in season in the autumn, when they are best to enjoy, and can be found in many varieties from sour to sweet or a combination in between.

Cabbage, Cauliflower, and Broccoli

Cruciferous vegetables offer a delicious flavor and texture, and can often grow in colder climates, making them easy to find in many regions. They are a good source of fiber, vitamins C, A and K, and iron. They can be enjoyed in a wide variety of dishes, including casseroles, stews, skillet meals, and soups. They are also great for salads in the raw and can be easily shredded and sprinkled over many dishes.

Foods to Avoid on the Paleo Diet

Which foods are best to avoid? For beginners to this diet, it may seem a bit challenging to determine which foods are Paleo-friendly and those that do not fit within this way of eating. Consider the types of foods that were available in primal times, when our ancestors hunted and gathered food, when there was no farming, cultivating, or harvesting done. Like every diet and healthy way of eating, Paleo encourages eating a wide range of whole, natural foods, without the need to count calories or worry about carbohydrates. In following this way of eating, it is imperative to include a wide range of foods that fit within the paleo criteria, while avoiding many other options that will negatively impact your progress. The types of foods that would not be around back then include the following, which are generally not included in the Paleo diet are as follows:

Grains and Legumes

Grains such as oats, wheat, barley, and bran are produced through farming, and for this reason, they are not included in the Paleo diet. Legumes are also farmed or harvested, and not included, as they were not part of the primal diet. Whole grains are a significant part of many meal plans; the Paleo diet easily replaces them with nuts, seeds, greens, and root vegetables.

Bread and Pastries

Bread and pastries are skipped completely on the Paleo diet. This is due to the amount of refined wheat, grains and ingredients used. Pastries are often full of sugar and glazes full of sweeteners and food coloring. Savory pastries may seem like a better option, with fewer sweeteners, though the ingredients include wheat flour that contains a lot of carbohydrates that convert into glucose in the body. Other items in rolls and savory treats may include smoked cheese and meat products, and other processed foods that should be excluded from your diet. If you have a bread craving, some excellent Paleo-friendly recipes include the replacement of wheat, dairy, and sugar ingredients for a better balance in the recipe.

Refined Sugars and Artificial Sweeteners

Any refined or unnatural sugars or sweeteners are completely avoided, and instead, natural sources such as maple syrup, agave, low carb (natural) options, and fruit (which contain fructose) are healthy options for sweetening desserts and drinks. Many pastries and baked goods contain refined sugar and preservatives, which should be avoided, as they can easily spike glucose levels. Artificial sweeteners are often used in place of sugar, which may seem like a good substitute. However, they are full of chemicals and artificial ingredients that can increase other risks to your health. If you want to avoid sugar completely, choose monk fruit or stevia, both of which are natural, sweet and have no impact on increasing blood sugar levels.

Trans Fats and Highly Processed Foods

Deep-fried foods and meals high in trans fats are completely avoided, due to their negative effects on health, and unnatural composition. These foods are responsible for increasing the likelihood of cancer, heart disease, and many other chronic conditions and disorders. Switching French fries for a baked root vegetable or salad is a good option for Paleo, as well as skipping the deep-fried chicken and burgers for a roast, baked, or lightly sautéed version. Onion rings, a popular fast food side, can be reinvented as a baked snack. Zucchini, kale, and pickles can be fried, baked or enjoyed as are in salads or as snacks.

Lot Fat or Zero Fat Foods

Food products labeled as fat-free or having zero fat are not included in the Paleo diet, due to their negative effects on the health. Examples of these foods include packaged cookies, crackers, and dairy products such as flavored yogurt and artisan cheeses. It is best to buy a plain, unsweetened, full-fat version of these foods instead of their artificially sweetened and flavored counterparts, which contain artificial colors, flavors, and hidden sugars. Many "fat-fee" or "low fat" foods are not effective in weight loss either and they are often unable to adequately satisfy hunger.

In general, all foods that are unnatural and include artificial ingredients can be skipped. If in doubt, read labels and choose options from the produce section of the grocery store or farmer's market as often as possible. Skip the grain and legumes aisle completely, and focus on adding root vegetables, in-season fruits, and other vegetables as your main and side features. Meat and dairy are best chosen as organic and with little or no additives. Include as many nuts and seeds as possible, and avoid any varieties with added sugars, coatings or sodium, even if the label promises they are natural. Dried fruits are a good option for a Paleo diet, as long as they are naturally sun-dried instead of chemically dried, which is common. For best options, buy your dried fruits in natural food stores or farmers' markets, where they are from a more natural source or homemade.

The Modified Version of the Paleo Diet

If you are looking for a slight variation from the original Paleo diet, either to gradually follow a full Paleo version or remain with a modified diet, this is a good option. Many people struggle with eliminating certain foods from their diet that are not conducive to Paleo eating. This may be due to having certain allergic restrictions or not being able to access certain foods within their region or immediate area that are Paleo. Easing the restrictions on the Paleo diet is a good way to improve your way of eating, by choosing low glycemic foods and avoiding processed goods, while maintaining decent eating habits. Consider the following criteria for the modified version of the Paleo diet:

- Grass-fed dairy is permitted, and if possible, choose unpasteurized as well. This variety of diary contains no preservatives and is more beneficial for your health as a result. Many farmer's markets, local farms, and some natural food stores may offer this variety of dairy.
- Certain grains and legumes are acceptable to include in a modified Paleo diet, as long as they are soaked, such as beans, to remove some of the additives or phytic acid that are present. By removing these, the beans and other grains become easier to digest. Fermented soybean products, such as miso and tempeh, are good options to include in your diet as well. They are rich in protein, calcium, and B12, and during the fermentation process, the common side effects of soy are removed, which often cause bloating and indigestion for some people. Brown rice, quinoa, buckwheat, and millet are good choices to include, as these grains contain high levels of nutrients. Other grains and

legumes can be enjoyed in moderation, though they should be organic and consumed with other sources of protein, calcium, and fiber.

- Choose gluten-free as much as possible. For example, if you choose to include a small portion of oats in your modified diet, choose gluten-free and organic as much as possible. You may want to include a handful of oats in a bowl of stewed apples with cinnamon, or with a coconut-based yogurt (or grass-fed dairy yogurt).

- Choose coconut oil as much as possible, and include in your daily meals and smoothies, drinks. MCT is the fat extract from coconut oil and can be added as well. The taste is neutral, which makes it an easy addition to many foods and drinks. Other healthy fats to include in your diet include avocado (and avocado oil), olive oil, and sesame oil. Nuts and seeds are also high in good fats and contribute to a balanced diet. These are an important part of the regular Paleo diet and should be included as regularly as possible.

- Root vegetables are a good source of energy and nutrients, though not all varieties are included in the regular Paleo diet, such as potatoes. Sweet potatoes (yams), beets, turnips, and other roots vegetables are good sources of fiber and satisfying in terms of taste and texture. Many of the dishes and recipes you can make with potatoes can be modified to include sweet potato fries or mashed, shredded turnips for hash browns or bakes in the oven, and roasted beets or fries. These types of vegetables allow for a lot of flexibility and options to spice and flavor. You can add them as a side dish or as a main meal. They are great to serve with a steak or serving of roast chicken or salmon.

Modified Paleo embodies the same principles of the regular Paleo, with a few changes to make it easy for people who may need to include a larger variety of foods that work best for their individual dietary needs. This includes diets that are vegan or plant-based and need the B12 and plant proteins that are contained in fermented soy foods. People who have an intolerance to gluten or wheat products may still want to include some legumes or gluten-free grain options in their diet for energy.

SIMPLE RECIPES FOR PALEO FOR BEGINNERS

BREAKFAST AND MID-MORNING Snacks

The first meal of the day is the most important fuel to begin your day. Breakfast is often skipped due to rushing off to work or daily errands, and while this is necessary sometimes, it can become a habit that can contribute to deficiencies and fatigue, which may hit by the late morning or early afternoon. These breakfast recipes are easy to prepare and include items that can be found at your local market or grocery store.

Poached Eggs and Asparagus

*P*repared poached eggs eliminate the need for cooking oils and a messy start, which may happen if you're in a rush. Simply poaching two eggs while lightly sautéing or steaming asparagus can be done together, while the coffee or tea is brewing. It may take a few tries to coordinate a few items at once, especially if you're focusing on getting your household ready, it can be easier to cook the poached eggs along with the asparagus in the same cooking pot. Seasoning for this dish includes sea salt and black pepper, though it can include paprika or a light dusting of parmesan cheese. Fresh asparagus is best, though cooking from frozen or preparing the night before (or from leftovers) is a quicker alternative to save time in the morning.

- ½ bunch of asparagus
- 2 teaspoons of butter
- 2 eggs
- Sea salt and black pepper
- Paprika (optional)

Boil 3 cups of water with sea salt and add in the asparagus, if uncooked, steaming for 10 minutes until almost tender, then drop one egg in at a time, poaching both for 5-10 minutes. The longer the eggs are poached, the harder the yolk, or softer and runny, if cooked less. Determine your preference and prepare the eggs while keeping an eye on the asparagus. Gently scoop the poached eggs onto a plate, while the asparagus is removed by draining the remaining water, and arrange on a plate, with butter, salt, and pepper, then top with the poached eggs. Sprinkle with paprika and parmesan cheese to serve.

Breakfast Patties With the Works

These patties are topped with a couple of layers of delicious ingredients, including eggs, avocadoes, and green peppers. The base is created with lean ground beef or pork or can sausage patties. For best results, prepare the patties home-made in a skillet, by forming them with the following ingredients:

- ½ pound of lean ground beef or pork

- 2 tablespoons of almond flour
- Pinch of sea salt, chili pepper, and black pepper
- 1 egg

Combine the ingredients in a bowl and form into patties, about 3" in diameter. Saute in a skillet heated with olive oil or butter, and fry on both sides until well done, then place on a plate. In the same skillet, prepare the eggs by frying them sunny side up, or poach them separately, and saute the green pepper (either with the eggs or separately). Include the following ingredients:

- Black pepper
- 2 eggs
- 1 avocado, ripe
- Half of the green pepper, sliced into strips (lengthwise)
- 1 teaspoon of dried chilies
- Fresh green onion, diced
- Pinch of paprika

Mash the avocado and mix with lime juice, chili pepper, or crushed chilies and sea salt with black pepper. Spread onto each meat patty, then place the sautéed green peppers, followed by placing each egg on top. Sprinkle with fresh green onions and paprika and black pepper.

Paleo Crepes

These are a nice switch from eggs, and only require three main ingredients, though other items may be added as desired. This recipe creates a light, smooth textured crepe that can accommodate any variety of toppings, including fresh berries, sliced bananas, dark chocolate, cocoa powder and/or cinnamon.

Maple syrup is another excellent option and a popular choice for pancakes. All of these toppings are paleo-friendly.

- 1 cup of each flour: tapioca and almond (coconut flour can be replaced with half of the almond flour, for a combination of all three, if desired)
- Raw sugar or monk fruit (roughly 2 teaspoons)
- 1 cup of milk (coconut or nut-based milk is recommended; a dairy is also an option)
- Dash of vanilla extract (this ingredient is optional)

With butter or olive oil, heat a skillet to a moderate or medium temperature, and mix the flours and milk with the vanilla extract and sweetener in a bowl, using a whisk to blend thoroughly. Once the batter is smooth, pour 3 or 4-inch diameter portions, one at a time, onto the skillet and cook evenly on both sides, approximately for 2-3 minutes each. Serve with the toppings of your choice.

Spinach and Smoked Salmon Omelet

*I*f you're in the mood for a decadent treat for a weekend brunch or looking to make use of leftover smoked salmon in your refrigerator or freezer, this is an ideal option. Raw or frozen (precooked) spinach can be used in this recipe. If you choose to use fresh spinach, chop it finely after washing and rinsing the leaves thoroughly. Onions and garlic are excellent options to enhance the medley of flavors.

- 3 eggs
- 1 cup of frozen or finely chopped spinach
- ½ cup of diced smoked salmon
- Dash of paprika and black pepper

- Chili powder (optional)
- Fresh dill
- Olive oil for the skillet
- Crushed garlic cloves
- 2 tsp of finely diced or crushed onions

Whisk the eggs, then add in the remaining ingredients, mixing well, then pour onto a heated skillet with olive oil. Cook until the omelet is evenly done, then flip one half over for a minute, followed by flipping the full omelet. Serve garnished or topped with fresh dill or chives.

Mushroom and Ham Omelet

*T*his omelet provides a wealth of protein, calcium, and healthy fats in one meal, and is ideal if you are ready for a busy day at work, or a vigorous exercise at the gym. This dish is low in carbohydrates, which accelerates the metabolism first thing in the morning. If you prefer this type of meal later in the day, it is a great option for lunch or as a light dinner, depending on your schedule. Any variety of mushrooms can be used. Cooked ham sliced into cubes, from a leftover roast, is ideal. If you have leftover roast ham, beef or other red meats in your refrigerator, they can be added to this omelet for a hearty breakfast or brunch.

- 3 eggs
- 1 ½ cups of cooked ham or beef, sliced into cubes or small pieces
- Black pepper and sea salt
- Dill, dried or fresh
- Fresh chives or grated onion, about 2 tablespoons
- Paprika, about 1 teaspoon

- Dash of chili pepper (optional)
- Olive oil
- Thinly sliced mushrooms, about ½ cup

Whisk the three eggs into a bowl, then add in the mushrooms, cubed meat, seasoning, and spices, including onion or chives, and other spices as desired. Heat a skillet with the olive oil, and gently pour in the egg mix to cook evenly for about 2-3 minutes. When the one side is cooked, lift half and fold over to the other, then gently flip and cook for another 2-3 minutes or until well done. Serve with a slice of Paleo bread, fresh greens or fruit salad.

Fruit Salad for Breakfast

*W*hether you enjoy a full breakfast with fruit on the side, or a simple bowl of fruit to get started, this is an ideal option to consider in the morning, or as a mid-morning snack. The fruits you choose for this salad are plenty, though it is best to pick foods in season, as they are fresh and easy to find at local markets. There are many fruits available year-round as well, whether fresh or frozen, including berries, mangoes, bananas, apples, and kiwi. If you decide to include fruits only available frozen, allow them to defrost at least one hour before adding to the recipe. If you pick apples for your fruit salad, add a little lemon juice to them to prevent them from turning brown, which can happen quickly.

- 1 ½ - 2 cups of fresh berries (blackberries, strawberries, blueberries, currants and/or raspberries)
- 1 sliced banana
- 2 kiwis, sliced
- 1 cup of sliced mango or pineapple chunks

- Sliced apple (1 small or medium)
- Orange or mandarin pieces (8-10)
- Fresh lemon juice

Combine the above ingredients into a large bowl and sprinkle lemon juice, freshly squeezed, over the fruits. Serve as a side with poached or fried eggs, or with a dollop of grass-fed yogurt.

Fried Eggs With Bacon and Spinach

A traditional breakfast, eggs, and bacon can be enjoyed as a weekend brunch or during the week. The best way to prepare bacon and minimize fried oils and grease is to bake them in the oven before preparing the eggs and spinach. Frozen spinach is a convenient option, as it is already cooked, and compressed into serving sizes. The equivalent of ½ cup of spinach is usually one serving in a frozen package of spinach. Alternatively, if you use fresh spinach, this can be served as a side with a light vinaigrette dressing.

- 1 cup of fresh or ½ cup of cooked spinach
- 3 eggs
- 4 slices of bacon
- Olive oil
- Sea salt and black pepper
- Paprika

Set the bacon in the oven on a baking tray, lightly greased with olive oil. Bake for 8-10 minutes, then monitor until crispy, at 350 degrees, then remove to cool. Prepare the eggs on a skillet with olive oil, and fry over-easy. Toss in the spinach, if cooked, or if raw, toss in a bowl with lemon vinaigrette. Serve the eggs over the spinach with the bacon on the side. Sprinkle sea salt, black pepper, and paprika on top. Serve over the spinach (raw or cooked) and add the bacon. If desired, crumble the bacon and sprinkle over the eggs. Paleo bread can be served with this meal, or a sliced grapefruit or orange.

Egg Breakfast Bites

*J*f you are looking for a breakfast-to-go option that can be prepared the night before, consider making these small, bite-sized breakfast treats that can be easily microwaved or reheated to go in the morning. All you need is a muffin tray, silicone or paper cups, and a few ingredients:

- 6 eggs, large (or 7-8 medium or small eggs)
- ½ cup of shredded sharp cheddar (unpasteurized and grass-fed)
- 2 tablespoons of crumbled crispy bacon or bacon bits
- 1 tablespoon of chives, finely chopped
- Sea salt and black pepper
- Paprika
- Chili pepper (or crushed dried chilies)

Whisk all the eggs in a large bowl, and toss in the paprika, sea salt, and black pepper. Add in the chives, chili pepper (optional), crispy bacon and shredded cheddar, and combine until all ingredients are evenly mixed. Pour into 6 silicone or paper muffin cups lining a tray, then place it in a preheated oven. Bake for approximately 12-14 minutes or until the egg cups are well done, then remove from the oven and serve after cooling for a few minutes. These breakfast bites can be refrigerated and enjoyed up to 3 days or added to the freezer for up to one month. Several batches can be prepared at once by doubling or tripling the recipe contents. Other ingredients to consider for this recipe:

- Cubed or shredded pieces of cooked ham
- Sliced and sautéed mushrooms (cook first, then add to egg cups)
- Lightly sautéed garlic or garlic powder
- Fresh parsley or dill, shredded, or dried

Lunch and Light Meals

Whether you enjoy a mid-morning snack in between breakfast and lunch or skip right to the middle meal of the day, it's important to include a good source of nutrients to boost your energy levels, which may be spent since the morning. Since rice, pasta, and grains are not used as a base for Paleo dishes, root vegetables, dark greens, and sprouts are often a good choice. Like low carb and ketogenic diets, paleo dishes may include "riced" or finely grated cauliflower or broccoli in place of rice, or spiral yams or zucchini instead of wheat pasta.

Beef or Poultry Bone Broth

*R*ecently, the health benefits of collagen and nutrient contained in beef and poultry bones have become popularly enjoyed as a broth. While common beef, chicken and vegetable broths are available in stores, a bone broth requires deep saturation of bones stewed in boiling water for at least 20-24 hours. The best way to obtain bones for preparing your home-made broth is by visiting your local butcher for leftover bones from cuts of meat, or the remainder of roast beef, turkey or chicken dinner. Other meat bones such as pork and venison can be used, though poultry and beef are the most common and popular in the Paleo diet. To prepare, add the bones of one carcass to 6-8 cups of water and boil until bubbling. Continue to boil for at least half an hour, then reduce and stew for another hour on moderately low. After this point, you can continue stewing the bones on low heat, adding your desired medley of spices, including sea salt, black pepper, savory, thyme, sage, chili powder, etc. Cover and stew on low for several hours. If you need to leave the area, turn the stove off completely and cover it until the next day. Remove from the stove after a total of 20-24 hours and use it as desired.

Ingredients for bone broth:

- Bones of one carcass or meal (1 chicken, turkey or roast beef)
- Sea salt
- Black pepper
- Desired spices and seasoning: chili pepper, thyme, oregano, savory, etc.

Bone broth can be stored in the refrigerator in a jar or resealable container for up to one week, or the freezer for up to 3 months.

Skillet Cauliflower and Bacon Crumble

*a*n aromatic and delicious vegetable, cauliflower is a mild, yet textured and tasty vegetable that combines well with many ingredients and flavors. This dish is easy to prepare and includes the addition of crumbled, crispy bacon that is best to prepare first or kept from breakfast or lunch leftovers. If you plan on making this dish and decide to include bacon with your breakfast, fry some extra to prepare for this meal in advance.

- 1 head of cauliflower, sliced into small florets, about 2-3 cups
- Butter, unsalted, for the skillet (olive oil can also be used)
- ½ or ¾ cups of bacon crumble
- Parmesan cheese, grated or dried
- Crushed garlic cloves, about 2 (finely diced or garlic powder)
- Sea salt and black better
- Paprika

Melt the butter in the skillet with the garlic, sea salt, pepper, and paprika. Saute for 2-3 minutes on moderate heat, before tossing in the cauliflower florets. Continue to cook, coating the cauliflower florets, sautéing them continuously until they are coated and lightly golden. Add in the parmesan cheese, approximately 2-3 teaspoons, and more butter, if needed. When the cauliflower is nearly done, fold in the bacon crumble and continue to stir lightly for a few minutes, then serve. Top with additional parmesan and/or parsley, if desired.

Skillet Portobello Mushrooms With Onions

*P*ortobello mushrooms are a nutrient-rich food that can be enjoyed as a main meal feature with onions, spices and other vegetables that can be tasty in a skillet. This dish is easy to create, using olive or avocado oil with fresh portobello mushroom caps.

- Portobello mushroom caps, 4 in total
- Olive oil
- Sea salt and black pepper
- Chili powder or dried chilies

- Paprika
- Sliced onion, 1 medium or large

Place the portobello mushroom caps in a heated skillet with olive or avocado oil and saute for a few minutes on each side. Toss in the onion slices, and saute once the mushrooms are nearly done, cooking them together. Top with the seasoning and spices, then serve with salad or as a light meal.

Lettuce and Tuna Wraps

*B*read and whole wheat wraps are not included in the Paleo diet, though lettuce wraps can substitute well, and provide a good option for holding a lot of ingredients and toppings. Canned tuna is convenient and best to use for this meal, though baked tuna is another option, especially if it is leftover from a previous dinner. Combine tuna with the following ingredients and add into a large lettuce leaf:

- 1 can of tuna, drained (water-based, not oil)
- Olive oil
- Chopped onion, about 2 tablespoons
- Chili powder
- Sea salt and black pepper

Drain the tuna from the can, and mash into a bowl with the olive oil, onion, and chili powder. Add in the sea salt and black pepper, and some of the following ingredients, as desired:

- Dried parsley or dill
- Chives, fresh or dried
- Mashed avocado

- Dash of lime or lemon juice

Scoop the mixture onto the lettuce leaf, then wrap and enjoy. This recipe will make approximately two leaf wraps.

Cucumber, Tuna and Arugula Salad

*L*ike tuna salad wraps, this recipe uses the same recipe as above and combines it with chunkier cuts of vegetables for a salad dish. This can be easily enjoyed as a full lunch on its own, or with soup. This salad contains major ingredients that are required in everyday meals, including protein, fiber, calcium, and vitamins. While the recipe includes cucumbers and arugula, there are many other ingredient possibilities available to change the flavor of this dish.

- Can of tuna, drained
- 1 small shallot, diced
- ½ cucumber (large) or a small cucumber, sliced into small ½-inch pieces
- 1 cup of arugula, diced
- Sea salt and black pepper
- Chili pepper (optional)
- Olive oil
- Lemon juice
- Dill or parsley (or both), dried or freshly chopped

Combine all the ingredients in a bowl, beginning with the tuna, mixing with the olive oil, sea salt, black pepper, lemon juice, chili pepper, and dill or parsley. Add in the cucumber and arugula, once the other ingredients are well combined, then serve.

Paleo Bread

. . .

*S*ince grains and baked goods are avoided on the Paleo diet, it can be challenging to find the alternative. This bread recipe is perfect for Paleo, as it contains only the diet-friendly ingredients, avoiding all grains and dairy. This is a loaf that can be created in your oven at home for any occasion and creates an excellent style of bread for any sandwich you choose to make.

- Almond Flour, 2 cups
- Coconut Flour, 2 tablespoons
- Baking soda, about 1 teaspoon
- Flaxseed meal or ground flax seeds, about ½ cups
- Arrowroot or tapioca flour, about ½ cup
- Baking powder, about 1 tablespoon
- Dash of sea salt
- 1/8 cups of almond or cashew milk
- 2 egg whites
- 3 large eggs
- 1 teaspoon of apple cider vinegar
- Coconut oil, about ¼ cups

Mix all the dry ingredients listed above in a large bowl, then set aside. Whisk the egg whites (2) in one bowl, and separately, the whole eggs (3) in another bowl. Stir in the dry mixture with the wet, and add in the almond or cashew milk, apple cider vinegar, coconut oil and eggs (egg whites and whole eggs). Move all the batter to a prepared baking loaf and set inside a preheated oven. Bake for 30 minutes or until loaf is done. This bread can be stored up to one week in the refrigerator.

Dinner Recipes

The final meal of the day doesn't have to be elaborate or time-consuming to be healthy and reasonable. Dinners can be a simple feast for one or two or a combination of several dishes and options for a family or larger household or group of people. The options in this section include both features of the main meal and the sides. These can be mixed and matched depending on your preference, and whether you prefer to include meat as a feature or more plant-based options. Many foods, both meat-based, and vegetables, can be prepared easily in the oven or skillet.

Baked Salmon With Dill and Parsley

*J*f you're a fan of salmon, one of the healthiest fish options to include in your diet, this dish is easy to prepare in the oven as you create side dishes. Frozen or fresh salmon steaks are ideal for this recipe, which are simply baked in a dish for 45 minutes with lemon juice and seasoning, and served with fresh lemon, dill, and parsley.

- Lemon juice (for coating the salmon steaks)
- 3-4 salmon steaks
- Black pepper, sea salt, fresh or dried dill
- Fresh parsley
- Olive oil (or avocado oil)
- Paprika and thyme

Coat the salmon steaks lightly in lemon juice, and place in a baking dish or tray lightly greased with olive oil or avocado oil. Coat lightly in seasoning (black pepper, sea salt, thyme, and paprika) and bake in the oven for 45-50 minutes at 350 degrees. Check periodically and remove once the fish is flaky and well done. Serve with additional fresh squeezed lemon juice, and garnish with dill and parsley. Serve with fresh arugula or spinach and/or ripe avocado as aside. A roasted root vegetable is another excellent option to serve with salmon.

Chicken Kale and Garlic Skillet

*T*his is an easy and quick skillet dish to make with chicken breast, garlic, kale and sesame oil with your choice of seasoning and spices. In this recipe, dried chilies, garlic powder, and cumin are recommended. For a savory taste, without heat, try combining savory, sage, thyme, and oregano combined. Chicken is versatile and provides an excellent source of lean protein. Sesame seeds are a great option as a topping for this dish, either raw or toasted.

- 1 pound of boneless, skinless chicken breast (organic is recommended)
- 3 cups of finely diced or shredded kale, with stems, removed
- Crushed garlic (grated or crushed, about 3 cloves)
- Sesame oil for frying
- Dried chilies or powder
- Black pepper and sea salt
- Dry roasted or raw sesame seeds
- Additional seasoning/spices to consider savory, thyme, oregano, etc.

Cut the boneless chicken into one-inch pieces, or slightly larger, and add to a skillet with sesame oil. Cook at a moderate temperature for 5-6 minutes, then toss in the garlic and spices. Continue to saute until chicken is well done, then reduce heat to low and toss in shredded kale. In another skillet, lightly toast the sesame seeds on moderate to high heat for 1-2 minutes, then set aside (raw sesame seeds can be used without toasting). Serve the sauteed chicken, garlic, and kale with spices sprinkled with sesame seeds on top.

Roasted Yams

*a*n excellent side dish, or as the main feature of a plant-based meal. Yams or sweet potatoes are excellent sources of vitamin A and fiber and can be easily prepared in the oven, much like regular potatoes. To prepare yams, scrub and wash them vigorously, then slice them in 3 or 4-inch pieces and add to a roasting pan. They usually take anywhere between 45-60 minutes to roast fully, and this timeframe should be taken into consideration when preparing other dishes or sides to serve together so that they are all done at the same time. Roasting yams in a medium pan or baking dish include the following simple ingredients:

- 3-4 yams or sweet potatoes (sliced into smaller pieces, about 3 or 4-inches in size)
- Paprika, thyme, sea salt, and black pepper
- Olive oil or butter
- Fresh parsley
- Sour cream (full fat, unsweetened). Plain Greek or Icelandic yogurt can also be used in place of sour cream

Prepare the baking tray or dish by coating with a thin layer of butter or olive oil, and place the yams inside, lightly sprinkling with olive oil or butter, sea salt, and the remaining spices. If some heat is desired, add a dash of cayenne, chili pepper, and/or Cajun spice. Bake, covered, in the oven for approximately 45-60 minutes, checking every 30 minutes on the progress. Depending on the oven and the size of the potatoes, the baking may take more or less time. Once the yams are tender, remove from the oven and serve topped with fresh butter (at room temperature), a dollop of sour cream and a dash of paprika on top with fresh parsley.

Broccoli, Cheese and Bacon Crumble Bake

*T*his is a delicious casserole that combines the delicious taste of baked broccoli and a variety of cheeses of your preference of unpasteurized, grass-fed cheese. While the Paleo diet doesn't typically include diary, unpasteurized dairy can be an option. This recipe includes shredding and mixing any 3-4 varieties of cheese to mix and top with the broccoli. This provides an in-depth medley of cheese taste, which complements the vegetables well.

- 1 head of broccoli, sliced into small florets
- 3-4 cups of shredded cheese, any type, and varieties. (Sharp or old cheddar is recommended, along with mozzarella, gouda and/or Monterey Jack or Swiss cheese).
- Butter at room temperature or olive oil
- Sea salt, black pepper, and paprika
- Almond flour and parmesan cheese (for the topping)

Toss the broccoli floret pieces with the shredded cheese, mixing evenly, then pour into a lightly greased casserole dish (with butter or olive oil). Ensure the cheese and broccoli are combined evenly, so there are no areas with little or no cheese. Mix the sea salt, black pepper, and paprika in a bowl with the parmesan cheese and almond flour (about 1-2 teaspoons each for the almond flour and parmesan cheese), then sprinkle carefully and evenly over the top of the casserole, before placing in the oven. Bake at 350 degrees for approximately 35-45 minutes, until the top is a light golden or brown color, then remove to slice and serve.

If you don't have enough broccoli or would like to mix the vegetable with other options, consider creating in the same casserole with the addition of sliced carrots, cauliflower florets, and/or parsnips.

Paleo Chili

*T*raditionally, chili is made with beans and legumes, which is where this recipe differs significantly. Vegetables such as zucchini, celery, carrots, onions, and dark greens take the place of beans. Tomatoes and garlic, along with chili powder and spices remain in this dish, along with lean ground beef. If you want an interesting twist on this dish, consider switching the beef with lamb or pork, or combining two different types of meats. Alternatively, this chili can be created as a vegan dish by skipping meat completely.

- Lean ground beef, about 1 pound
- 2 teaspoons of chili powder
- Sea salt and black pepper
- Crushed or pureed tomatoes, about 4 cups
- Onion, about 1/2 cup diced
- Crushed garlic cloves or powder
- Celery, chopped, about 1 cup
- Zucchini, small or medium, diced
- Carrots, diced
- Mushrooms, sliced thinly
- Olive oil for sauteing the beef

*A*dd the beef or lean ground meat of your choice to a heated skillet with olive oil, and cook well until brown, then add the onions, garlic, spices, and saute for a few more minutes, at a moderate temperature. Add all the vegetables and continue to cook. Saute until the vegetables are tender, then add the contents of the skillet to a large cooking pot to begin stewing the chili. Cook on low or a slightly moderate to low temperature, stirring in the tomato sauce, additional spices and if desired, more tomato sauce or diced tomatoes. Serve in a bowl as a main dish or light lunch.

Chicken Breast Skillet Meal With Greens

*T*his is a delicious meal with slices of chicken breast marinated with sesame seed oil and spices, cooked with a handful of spinach and kale, or an assortment of greens, including broccoli, arugula and/or cabbage. This skillet meal is highly nutritious and ideal for a boost of energy for later in the day. Ideally, if there is enough food left, you can set aside a portion or two for leftovers the next day. If desired, set aside for up to 3-4 days in the refrigerator. Skillet meals with meat tend to marinate more after at least one day, allowing the various flavors included to saturate and strengthen the taste.

- 2 chicken breast, boneless, cut into smaller, bite-sized pieces
- Sesame oil, to marinate the chicken
- Olive oil, for the skillet
- 1 cup of raw spinach

- Arugula, (approx. ½ cup), raw
- 1 cup of diced broccoli florets
- 1 cup of shredded cabbage
- 1-2 cups of other vegetables, as desired
- Sesame seeds, about 1 tablespoon
- 2 teaspoons of orange juice and zest
- Crushed garlic cloves, about 1-2
- Shredded or grated onion, about ¼ cup

*N*ote: it is ideal to marinate the chicken in sesame oil and orange juice overnight, to strengthen the taste before adding to the skillet.

*T*he skillet is prepared by adding the olive oil and placing the chicken pieces inside. After a few minutes, add in the onion, garlic, and seasoning, sautéing for another 8-10 minutes, until the chicken is tender, and the spices and ingredients added so far are saturated into the chicken. If there is any sesame oil or orange zest or juice are leftover from marinating, or no margination is done before this dish, add into the skillet as the chicken is cooking with the spices. After a few minutes, add in the remaining ingredients and simmer at a moderate temperature until all the ingredients are tender. Serve sprinkled with sesame seeds.

Cashew Beef, Asparagus, and Chili Peppers

*S*tewing beef is ideal for this recipe, or a similar cut of beef sliced into one or two-inch pieces. Cashews offer an excellent layer of texture and taste to a sautéed dish of beef with asparagus and olive oil. Chili pepper is used to spice the plate as the beef is cooked. The asparagus takes a while to cook and can either be steamed before adding to the skillet, or adding in sooner, as the beef is cooking.

- 1 pound of beef, sliced into cubes
- 1 cup of coarsely chopped cashews, or whole (these can be dry roasted)
- Chili peppers, dried or in powder form
- ½ bunch of asparagus, sliced in half
- Olive oil
- Crushed garlic cloves

*T*oss the cubed beef into a prepared skillet with olive oil and saute for a few minutes, then add in the garlic, chili pepper, and asparagus. The beef will take a while to cook, as will the asparagus, which can either be sautéed in the same skillet or separately. Cook for at least 15-18 minutes, then serve with lightly dry roasted cashews as a topping.

Lamb Burgers

*T*hese are a tasty meal option that can be enjoyed with any variety of fresh toppings, including caramelized onions and greens. Ground lamb is the ideal option, though beef or chicken are also options (these recipes can be found below).

. . .

round lamb, 1 pound

Almond flour, 1/2 cup

1 egg

Tarragon, 1 teaspoon

Sea salt and black pepper

Dill or parsley, dried or fresh and diced

Olive oil

se the olive oil to heat the skillet to a moderate temperature, while preparing the ingredients in a bowl. Combine the ground lamb, egg, sea salt, black pepper, parsley, and tarragon. Mix well until all ingredients are evenly distributed, then form burger patties and fry individually on the skillet, about 3-5 minutes on each side. Serve on a lettuce leaf or as is, with some of the following toppings:

uacamole, freshly made, or sliced avocado

Sliced tomatoes

Fresh or caramelized onions

Fresh spinach or arugula

Pesto

Fresh dill or parsley

Mustard

Black olives, pitted and sliced

Jalapeno pepper

Chicken Meatballs

*T*his dish is baked in the oven with tomato sauce and a combination of spices and seasoning. Beef or pork can be substituted when chicken is unavailable.

*G*round chicken, lean, about 1 pound

1 teaspoon of garlic powder

Sea salt and black pepper

Olive oil

Savory spice

Paprika

Thyme

1 egg

1/4 cup of almond flour

*I*n a large bowl, combine the ground chicken with the egg, sea salt, black pepper, and seasoning. Mix well, then add in the almond flour, combining evenly. Form the mixture into 1-inch balls or one and a half-inch in diameter, then place on a prepared baking sheet. Bake in the oven at 350 degrees for 35-45 minutes, until done, then serve with your choice of tomato sauce.

Garlic Shrimp With Spinach and Lemon

$\mathcal{T}$his is an ideal dinner option if you have shrimp in the freezer. This is a simple meal that doesn't require a lot of preparation and can be prepared in a matter of minutes. Spinach tends to shrink when it is cooked, and for this reason, two cups or one bunch of spinach is good for a sizable serving. One pound of shrimp is ideal, and in large size, though a slightly larger or smaller serving will work for this recipe. The feature of this meal is the garlic and spices used to enhance the experience.

- 1 pound of shrimp (large, jumbo shrimp) or medium in size
- Crushed cloves of garlic (about 2-3)
- Dill, dried or fresh
- Olive oil
- Sea salt and black pepper
- 2 cups of raw spinach, washed and trimmed
- Sliced mushrooms (optional)

Olive oil is used to heat the skillet to medium, then add in the shrimp. If cooking from frozen, allow enough time to cook thoroughly, about 8-10 minutes, then add in the garlic, black pepper, sea salt, and dill. Add in the spinach and cook on moderate, ensuring all the leaves are fully cooked, and begin to shrink. Toss in the mushrooms, when the shrimp and spinach are almost done, then cook for a couple of more minutes, before removing to serve with sliced lemon.

Other options to consider for this recipe include:

- Adding roasted or raw almonds to the stir fry or skillet, when preparing this meal
- A dash of crushed chili peppers
- Fresh paprika, sprinkled on the dish to serve
- Leftover, cooked chicken breast from a roast or previous stir fry

Meal Replacements and Smoothies

Life is busy for most people, which makes preparing a full meal often challenging. If you encounter busy mornings or hectic schedules that don't allow for much meal planning, having a selection of snacks and go-to items to grab on your commute or errands.

Avocado and Coconut Milk Smoothie

*C*oconut and avocadoes contain a wealth of healthy fats, along with a good source of nutrients, including vitamins and fiber. This Smoothie combines the pleasant flavors of avocado and coconut with maple syrup or a low carb sweetener for a satisfying replacement for a quick drink.

- Coconut milk (1 cup)
- Avocado (ripened, soft)
- Maple syrup (1-2 tbsp)
- Coconut cream (optional)

Mix all the ingredients in a blender and pulse until the result is smooth. Serve immediately. As an option, add a banana with another cup of milk.

Mango and Kefir Smoothie

. . .

*M*angoes are a good source of vitamin A, C, and fiber. Combining them with kefir, a stronger fermented yogurt drink, is an ideal way to strengthen gut health and microbial balance in the body. Kefir can be found in grocery stores and natural food markets. It's best to choose plain, unsweetened and unflavored kefir, instead of the flavored options, which often include hidden sugars and artificial flavors.

- Mangoes (1 large or 2 small)
- 1 cup of kefir
- Coconut or almond milk (1 cup)
- Maple syrup or raw sugar

Mix the ingredients and blend for 40 seconds, then taste test and add more milk and/ or sweetener as needed. Continue to blend, then serve.

Peanut Butter and Chocolate Smoothie

*T*his smoothie combines the sweetness of chocolate with the protein and calcium richness of peanut butter. Cashew, almond or another nut butter can be used in place of peanut butter if desired. Smooth nut-butter is the best option without added sugar or sodium. The smooth texture mixes well with the cocoa or chocolate and blends easier in the food processor or blender.

- Coconut or almond milk (2 cups)
- Smooth, unsalted and sugar-free peanut butter (1 cup)
- ½ cup of melted chocolate or the equivalent in dark cocoa powder, unsweetened

- Maple syrup (1-2 tbsp)
- Coconut cream (optional)
- Dash of vanilla or almond extract

Mash the peanut butter and melted chocolate or cocoa powder together, then add in the sweetener, coconut cream, and vanilla or almond extract. Scoop into a blender and add in the two cups of coconut or almond milk, then pulse for 45-60 seconds, until smooth, then serve.

Banana and Pistachio Smoothie

*B*ananas are a powerful form of energy, providing a significant dose of fiber and potassium to any dish they are added. In a smoothie, their nutritional value is strong, as they are raw and enjoyed immediately. Pistachios are a tasty, green nut that pairs well with the taste of bananas, providing additional protein, healthy fats, and calcium.

- 1 ripe banana
- ¼ cup of shelled, raw pistachios (without sodium or sugar)
- Dash of sea salt
- 2 cups of almond, dairy or coconut milk
- Dash of vanilla extract
- Maple syrup, agave or a low carb sweetener

Mash the ripe banana in a bowl with the vanilla extract, sweetener, and sea salt. In a grinder, blend the raw, shelled pistachios until they resemble a fine powder. Add into the bowl and mix, then scoop into a blender or food processor with the milk, and pulse for about 45-60 minutes, until smooth. Serve topped with a sprinkle of cardamom or cinnamon.

Almond Butter and Cocoa Cups

*T*he combination of almond and cocoa is not only delicious but healthy and full of nutrients. Dark chocolate contains antioxidants, while almond butter is a good source of protein, healthy fats, and calcium. These cups are prepared without the use of baking, and only require a small saucepan to melt the chocolate which can be done with coconut oil or grass-fed butter.

- ½ cup of smooth almond butter, preferably organic
- 6-8 squares of dark chocolate (baker's chocolate)
- 2 teaspoons of agave or maple syrup (low carb sweetener can also be used)
- 1 teaspoon of coconut oil or softened butter

To prepare for this recipe, add silicone or paper cups to a muffin tray. These cups contain three layers: chocolate on the top and bottom and almond butter in the center. The baker's chocolate is melted in a small saucepan on medium with coconut oil and sweetener at a low temperature to prevent burning. When the chocolate is completely melted, remove from the stove and cool for a few minutes. Gently scoop enough chocolate to fill ¼ or ½ inches at the bottom of each cup. Depending on the size of the cups, this may fill 6-8 muffin cups and should leave enough for the top layer. Place in the freezer for 15-20 minutes, which will allow the chocolate to harden. Remove after this time frame and scoop enough almond butter to fill about ½ inch for the second layer or center of each cup.

Return the muffin tray to the freezer for another 15-20 minutes, or until the almond butter has hardened. Remove to add the final layer of chocolate on top and return to the freezer for the final 15-

20 minutes. After the final set, the cups are immediately ready to serve. They can also be left in the freezer for longer, or transferred to the refrigerator, though should onlu6be removed when ready to enjoy, as they will quickly melt at room temperature. These snacks are also referred to as ketogenic or keto "fat bombs," as they contain a good portion of healthy fats and energy, with moderate protein. The keto version includes low carb sweetener, though, in Paleo, any natural, unrefined sugar or sweetener can be added.

Coconut Blueberry Cheesecake Cups

*T*his is a delicious treat that can be easily created using the same muffin tray arrangement like the above recipe. These cups provide the rich, satisfying taste of cheesecake without the sugars or artificial flavors. Full-fat, unsweetened or unflavored cream cheese is used for this recipe, including the addition of plain, shredded coconut and frozen or fresh blueberries.

- 2 cups of plain, unsweetened and unflavored cream cheese
- Fresh or frozen blueberries
- 2-3 tablespoons of shredded coconut (unsweetened)
- Pinch of vanilla extract
- 2-3 teaspoons of maple syrup, agave or low carb sweetener

Before using the cream cheese, ensure it is softened at room temperature. If using from the refrigerator, microwave for approximately 30-40 seconds, until it is softened, and easy to mix with other ingredients. Mash the cream cheese, shredded coconut, sweetener, and sweetener, and combine well, so there are no uneven chunks of ingredients, and none of the items are clumped together. Gently fold in the blueberries, and scoop into silicone or paper muffin cups, filling approximately 2/3 or ¾ full each. Set in the freezer for about 20-25 minutes, then serve. These treats are full of protein and fiber and make an excellent snack before the gym or in the summer during a quick dash outside to work or errands. Keep these cups in the refrigerator or freezer until serving, as they will melt at room temperature.

Coconut and Pineapple Smoothie

A tropical-themed recipe, this smoothie is refreshing and ideal during the summer months.

2 cups of coconut milk

1 cup of pineapple chunks, fresh or frozen

Raw sugar or maple syrup

Vanilla collagen protein powder (optional), 1 tablespoon

I n a blender, combine the ingredients and pulse for at least 40 seconds. Add more of the ingredients, if needed, or ice to this drink to cool down if the pineapple isn't frozen. Papaya or mango can be added as well, or used in place of the pineapple

Cocoa and Cashew Nut Smoothie

A rich-tasting smoothie and without dairy, this smoothie is a decadent combination of cashew milk, butter, and cocoa powder.

. . .

2 cups of cashew milk

Cocoa powder, about 2 tablespoons

Raw sugar or maple syrup

Cocoa or vanilla collagen powder (optional), 1 tablespoon

1 ripe banana, optional

*C*ombine all the ingredients and blend for 35-45 seconds, then serve.

Desserts

Sweets and treats can be enjoyed as part of a balanced Paleo diet, which includes a wide range of natural ingredients, including fruits, unrefined sweeteners, milk, cream, nuts, and seeds. These recipes are simple and tasty, without all the artificial and refined ingredients often found in the baked goods, pastries, puddings, and custards.

Vanilla and Raspberry Chia Seed Pudding

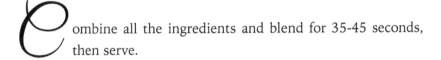

*T*his is a simple recipe to create with a few ingredients. Chia seeds are a rich source of many nutrients, including antioxidants, calcium, protein, and fiber. There are many variations of chia seed pudding recipes, including this basic vanilla flavor, with the addition of frozen or fresh raspberries. Chia seed puddings are best prepared the night before, as they "gel" with milk or yogurt overnight in the refrigerator, ready for enjoyment the following day.

- ¾ cups of chia seeds
- ½ cup of fresh or frozen raspberries
- Maple syrup or low carb sweetener
- 2 cups of milk (dairy or nut-based milk; coconut milk is another option)
- Dash of vanilla extract
- 2 teaspoons of cream, either dairy or coconut cream

Pour the milk and cream into a bowl and whisk together, while adding in the sweetener, vanilla extract, and chia seeds. Ensure all the ingredients are well combined before stirring in the raspberries. Refrigerate overnight, or for a minimum of two hours, then enjoy.

Chocolate Chia Pudding

*L*ike the recipe above, this tasty dish includes the infusion of rich, dark chocolate, which can be melted in advance or used in cocoa powder form, combined with coconut oil and natural sweetener. To melt chocolate, unsweetened baker's chocolate is the best option or another bar chocolate that is roughly 85-90% or more in cocoa content. The higher the percentage of cocoa, the more nutrient-dense the result, and less sugar.

- ¾ cups of chia seeds
- ½ bar of dark chocolate (baker's chocolate or cocoa powder)
- Maple syrup or low carb sweetener
- 2 cups of milk (coconut or nut-based milk; coconut milk is another option). Chocolate almond or nut-based milk is an option, though it's important to check if there are artificial sugars or flavors before including.

- 1-2 teaspoons of cocoa powder
- 2 teaspoons of cream, either dairy or coconut cream

Melt the baker's chocolate slowly on a low temperature in a saucepan with coconut oil and sweetener until the result is smooth without any lumps or clumps. Once this is achieved, remove from the stove, or keep on the burner and shut off the stove. Cool for a few minutes before adding to the coconut milk, cream, whisking thoroughly, then adding in the cocoa powder, chia seeds, and additional sweetener, if desired. Taste test to ensure the sweetness level is to your liking, and ensure the chia seeds are well mixed, then refrigerate overnight or for a couple of hours, then enjoy. When serving, top with dark chocolate chips or shavings.

Paleo Brownies

*I*t is possible to create a delicious baked recipe without processed wheat or grains. This recipe replaces whole wheat with tapioca flour and almond flour. Coconut oil is also used, along with coconut sugar, both of which are Paleo-friendly. These brownies are easy to prepare and bake in the oven within half an hour.

- Coconut oil, about ½ cup
- Dark chocolate chips, about 1 cup (chocolate shavings will also work)
- 3 tablespoons of cocoa powder
- Tapioca flour, about ½ cup
- Sea salt
- 3 eggs
- Vanilla extract

- Espresso powder (optional) or crushed coffee beans, about 1 teaspoon
- Almond flour or crushed almonds, 1 tablespoon

Melt the chocolate chips and coconut oil in a saucepan on low heat or in a microwave for 20 seconds. In a mixing bowl, add the coconut sugar, flours, eggs, sea salt, and espresso powder. Combine well, then blend with an electric or manual hand-held mixer for about one minute. Fold in the melted chocolate with coconut oil and use the mixer to combine evenly. Pour the batter into a prepared baking loaf pan and set inside a preheated oven to bake at 350 degrees for 25-30 minutes. Use a toothpick to determine when the brownies are done. Remove from the oven to cool for a few minutes, then slice and serve. Sprinkle flakes of sea salt on each brownie, if desired.

LIFESTYLE AND THE PALEO DIET

The Importance of Exercise

Staying active and getting enough exercise is one of the most important ways you can stay healthy with a balanced diet. This does not require athletic feats of movement or becoming a daily gym guest, though the more you work out, the better you will utilize the nutrients in a Paleo diet and use them to benefit your body overall.

Finding the Right Exercise and Dietary Routine for Long-term Results and Lifetime Benefits

Exercise and working out means something different to everyone. If you walk once a day for an hour, this may be enough for your ability and fitness level, whereas other people may engage in high impact sports or more strenuous exercise to achieve certain results. Different types of movement and activities that are important for a balanced lifestyle include the following:

- Yoga, stretching, and mindful mediation. This is a great way to relieve stress, realign your focus and increase your flexibility.
- Weight training and lifting are essential ways to build muscle and tone
- Aerobics and cardiovascular exercise are important for weight loss and overall toning. It's a great way to increase endurance and your fitness level
- Cycling, swimming, jogging, sprinting, and team sports are all examples of how to stay in shape. Also, dance lessons, martial arts, and tai chi are excellent options as well.

Bonus Recipes for On the Go

Do you need a quick snack or serving of nutrients and energy on the go? These recipes are ideal for making something in a pinch.

Crispy Kale Chips

*I*f you're looking for a healthy snack that can be prepared in a matter of minutes, this is an ideal option and requires just one bundle of kale with sea salt and olive oil (coconut oil or avocado oil can also be used.

- 3 cups of raw kale pieces, cut from a fresh bundle, into bite-sized portions
- Sea salt or pink Himalayan salt
- Olive oil (coconut oil or avocado oil are also options)

Lightly and evenly coat all the kale pieces with olive oil and place them on a baking tray. Parchment paper is recommended to ensure the kale does not stick to the tray when baking in the oven.

Sprinkle evenly and lightly with sea salt over the chips, then bake for 8-10 minutes at 375 degrees. Keep an eye on the oven for the first one or two attempts of this recipe. Due to the type of kale (curly, red, etc.), the cooking time may be more or less by a minute or two, and may burn quickly or not cook fully (this can change within just one minute, as kale is thin and cooks fast!).

There are a few options and variations to consider for kale chips if you want to add a twist to the flavor:

Cumin or Curry Flavored Kale Chips

Add a sprinkle of curry powder and/or cumin mixed with sea salt. The baking time should be approximately the same time frame as the regular recipe.

Parmesan Kale Chips

Add a light coating of dried, shredded parmesan cheese along with the sea salt. Black pepper is also a good option combined with the parmesan and salt. These chips may take another one or two minutes to cook fully, approximately 10-12 minutes, at a temperature of 375 degrees.

Spicy Kale Chips

Combining a dash of chili powder, cayenne pepper or Cajun spice is ideal for spicy kale chips. These will cook for about 8-10 minutes, roughly the same time frame as the regular chips.

Baked Onion Rings

These are a nice alternative to the deep-fried variety, which is full of trans fats and unhealthy ingredients. This recipe is easily made with several ingredients to coat the onion rings and bake them for 15-16 minutes in the oven at 350 degrees.

- 2 medium or 1 large red onion, sliced into rings
- 1 cup of almond flour
- 2 eggs
- Sea salt
- Cajun spice
- Black pepper

Mix the black pepper, sea salt, and Cajun spice in a bowl, then combine with the almond flour. This will serve as the coating on the onion rings. Whisk the two eggs in a separate bowl, and coat each onion ring thoroughly first, before coating with the almond and spice combination, and place on a prepared baking tray. Bake for approximately 15-16 minutes, until the onion rings are crispy, but not burnt. Serve with salsa or coconut-based sour cream dip or enjoy as is. These are an excellent snack in place of potato chips or popcorn.

Spicy Guacamole

*A*vocados are a great option for the Paleo diet, as they are high in fiber, healthy fats, and energy. Guacamole is a great side or dish to include with a variety of meals, as a side to chili or skillet meal, or as a burger topping.

- 2 avocadoes, ripe
- Olive oil, about 2 teaspoons
- Freshly squeezed lime juice
- Chili powder or cayenne
- Grated onion, about 2 tablespoons

- ½ a tomato, diced
- Black pepper and sea salt
- Fresh cilantro

Mash the fresh avocados in a bowl and add in the sea salt, black pepper, olive oil, lime juice, and spices. Combine well, and fold in the tomatoes and onions, ensuring they are mixed well. Top with cilantro to serve.

FREQUENTLY ASKED QUESTIONS

ONCE YOU BEGIN ADAPTING to the Paleo diet, you may have additional questions or concerns that can be addressed here. The following frequently asked questions provide more information on how to approach individual situations and customizing your way of eating Paleo.

Question: Can the Paleo diet be adapted for vegan and plant-based diets?

Answer: The Paleo diet can be adapted to fit a plant-based meal plan. However, there are key vegan foods that would not be Paleo friendlies, such as soy, edamame beans, legumes, and fermented versions of soy, such as miso and tempeh. Dairy products would be replaced with nut-based milk, yogurt, and butter, made from almond, peanut, cashews and coconut milk. Plant-based proteins appropriate for the Paleo diet include nuts, seeds, dark greens, and sea vegetables. It may be a challenge to incorporate Paleo into a vegan diet, though with adequate research and dedication, it is possible.

Question: Is there a limitation on the amount of sugar you can have when following the Paleo diet?

Answer: Sugar is not strictly forbidden or avoided, as long as it is fructose or another natural, unrefined source, such as agave or maple syrup. As long as your diet and food choices are predominantly natural and without processing, including meat and dairy products in their natural, unflavored form, there will be little concern for excessive sugar, as you will only receive the required amounts in each serving. In other words, eating a fully natural, organic diet provides a balance of all nutrients on its own, without the need to strictly monitor sugar.

Question: Are there any drawbacks to following a Paleo diet?

Answer: Generally, there are no risks in following a Paleo diet, as all the foods are natural and full of nutrients, without any processed or artificial ingredients. There have been some concerns about the chances of increasing the risk of heart disease, due to the number of fats in the Paleo diet, though there are no studies to support this concern, and in fact, Paleo has shown a positive impact on heart health and reducing the risk of heart conditions, due to the number of nutrients and fiber, and the lack of processed foods. Choosing this way of eating will significantly reduce your risk of many diseases and conditions associated with unhealthy food choices.

Question: Is dairy allowed on the paleo diet?

Answer: On a strict paleo diet, dairy is not included; however, some people may add it in small amounts. Some Paleo diets allow for milk, cheese, yogurt, and butter if they are from grass-fed animals, though generally it's limited or avoided. It's important to determine how much dairy you want to include, if at all, and check the source to confirm how likely it is to be a good option. Grass-fed is ideal and should be the standard for meat products as well. If you can access raw, unpasteurized milk, some Paleo diets accept this as an option because it is unprocessed, and the goal of this diet is to include whole foods as much as possible. Depending on where you live, unpasteurized milk may or may not be available, depending on the food guidelines and legislation in your region. If you want to add dairy, and are unable to find unpasteurized as an option, there are grass-fed milk products available in natural food stores as a good option.

Question: Is Paleo similar to the keto diet?

Answer: There are some similarities between keto and Paleo, where the level of protein is moderate, and healthy fats are included in place of high carb, processed foods. There are some important differences as well:

- The keto or ketogenic diet focuses on adjusting the fat content to be high, around 75% of the diet, followed by moderate amounts of protein and low levels of carbohydrates. On the other hand, Paleo doesn't follow strict guidelines for how much of each macronutrient to include, but rather, focuses on the types of foods and nutrient quality instead.
- The paleo diet includes many of the same types of foods as Paleo, without being specific in fat and protein content. While the focus of both diets interns of ow foods are chosen is different, the outcome is generally the same for weight loss and overall results.
- Both diets focus on including healthy sources of protein, either meat or plant-based, preferably from organic and grass-fed sources. While the Paleo diet doesn't actively include dairy products, except for grass-fed and unpasteurized options, the keto diet allows for more full-

fat dairy products, provided they do not contain additives, flavors, and sugars.

Question: *How long does it take to see the results of a Paleo diet?*

Answer: Like any new way of eating, it can take a few weeks to one month to notice a change. Paleo is a lifestyle approach to eating, focusing on the quality of food choices you make, rather than focusing on portions and restrictions. To see the results of the diet, keep your meals planning and indulges consistent with natural, whole foods, and avoid all processed options. If you add in a few grains or a dish with non-Paleo food now and again, it's understandable, especially if they were regular choices in your meals before beginning this way of eating. Take your time, and don't feel discouraged if you don't see the results you expect right away. For most people, results take about one or two months, though it can happen sooner. Overall, you will reap the benefits of eating and feeling better.

Question: *What is the purpose of the Paleo diet, and why was it developed?*

Answer: The Paleo diet was developed to return to a primal way of eating, which does not include foods that are the result of farming or processing. It is strongly believed that our way of eating and health fares much better with the hunting and gathering method, which is most compatible with our development and genetics. Removing foods from our diet that involve farming and processing, is how we can realign our march to an original diet. This can alleviate many of the health conditions and problems we face today, which can be avoided by eating primal.

Question: *Is the Paleo diet one of the best ways to eat?*

Answer: It is considered one of the healthiest ways to eat because it closely follows the way our ancestors ate, which is based on natural meats, fruits, vegetables, nuts, and seeds. It doesn't restrict calories or require fasting, two factors that can affect some people's physical reactions to the diet. Following a balanced, nutritious way of eating is one of the best ways to eat, which Paleo aims to achieve.

Question: Can I follow the Paleo diet, even if I have allergies or serious reactions to certain types of foods contained in the Paleo diet?

Answer: Yes, anyone can follow the Paleo diet, and any foods that cause a reaction can simply be avoided. Often, the foods that create allergic reactions are processed foods, dairy, or wheat products, all of which are not included in the Paleo diet, except for some unpasteurized milk products. Shellfish and nut allergies can be avoided by omitting these foods completely. Fortunately, Paleo can be customized to give you a lot of options, which include a wide range of fruits and vegetables.

Question: Are there restaurants that cater specifically to the Paleo diet?

Answer: With the increase in popularity, there are some diners and restaurants that offer a good variety of Paleo-friendly foods, or they may be open to modifying menu choices to accommodate them. In urban areas, you may find more specific niche cafes and food services for certain dietary needs, many of which can fit within Paleo, such as gluten-free, ketogenic, and grass-fed meat options. Some cafes offer take-out services and custom orders that fit within a wide range of dietary options, including Paleo.

Question: Do people generally follow a Paleo diet for the long term?

Answer: It varies depending on your individual goals, though most people can easily adapt to Paleo for many years. It is sustainable, includes food choices that are easy to find at grocery stores and markets. Once you notice and experience the advantages of the Paleo diet, you'll want to continue following it longer, as it can only make a positive impact on your life!

The Paleo diet is a way of eating that has captured the attention of many people worldwide, due to its many advantages and focus on nutrients. By enjoying a wide range of fresh fruits, vegetables, and lean meats, among many other food options, such as nuts and seeds, your body and health will reap the many benefits associated with good food choices and a sustainable, long-term lifestyle of eating and living well.

CONCLUSION

Tips, Suggestions for Success on the Paleo Diet

Now that you've begun your journey to living and eating the Paleo way of life, you will likely encounter situations where you're unsure of which foods items should be included. While the parameters are clear initially, many food options in stores are vague about their contents and hide as much about artificial ingredients and hidden sugars as they can. This raises a lot of concerns, especially when avoiding as many unnatural and unhealthy options as possible. To ensure your success on this diet, consider the following tips and suggestions:

- Choose fresh produce only, and shop for frozen in a natural state, where the fresh option of fruits and/or vegetables is not readily available. Frozen vegetables and fruits are a great alternative when the option you want is not in season or not available in the produce section. Avoid canned fruits, as they contain syrup and sugars, while canned vegetables and related sauces contain high sodium, and other artificial ingredients, including sugar.

- Meat and dairy quality are more important than quantity. Make the most of your neighborhood, and locate local butchers, farmer's markets and shops that provide good options. Some supermarkets offer local goods reflecting the community and may offer organic meats and/or cheese options in their deli. Choose fresh or frozen meats, and avoid processed meat slices, as they contain carcinogens and nitrates, both of which contribute to a higher risk or cancer and heart disease.

- Nuts and seeds tend to be expensive, especially if they are fresh and from a good source. If possible, buy in bulk, so that you can choose the portion and custom the types of nuts and seeds you prefer. Cashew and pistachios tend to be expensive, whereas walnuts, peanuts, almonds, and pecans are less costly.

- Create as many foods and meals from home as possible. There are plenty of grocery stores and restaurants that offer Paleo-friendly foods, which is helpful in a pinch and convenient. However, some store-bought items may not be as fitting within the Paleo diet as they claim. For this reason, read labels and ingredients on all the items before you purchase them, and beware of any claims that are not accurate. Save your wallet and your diet by knowing what to buy.

CPSIA information can be obtained
at www.ICGtesting.com
Printed in the USA
LVHW042352130420
653369LV00015B/1299

9 781087 876221